Professor Richard Dawkins' 'Therapy Session' With the Wonderful Counsellor

I0224023

Debra C. Rufini

chipmunkapublishing
the mental health publisher

Debra C. Rufini

Published by
Chipmunkapublishing
PO Box 6872
Brentwood
Essex CM13 1ZT
United Kingdom

http://www.chipmunkapublishing.com

Chipmunkapublishing gratefully acknowledge the support of Arts Council England.

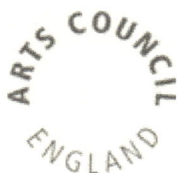

From the author

I pray that all who read this book will gain a blessing from it.

This faith of mine is the one that I share with my Brothers and Sisters who are spread out all over the world, but who are bound together as one through the shedding of the blood of the Lord Jesus Christ. So to my Christian family who I have not met as yet, may the Lord bless you and be ever with you as you continue to fight for him in his army. We are privileged to carry out this great task to reach for all those people who are so clearly carrying on with life regardless of him, its provider.

For those of you who read this book, who have not yet surrendered your all unto the King, my prayer is that your eyes will be opened and steered towards his guiding light, so that you too can be made whole in accepting him in, and become one in his family. He loves you.

I would like to thank my family, along with the many friends who have always been there when I have needed them. I value your friendship immensely. May the Lord richly bless you and protect you in his safe and secure keeping under his wing.

I dedicate this book to my Christian parents, John & Marie, who have raised me in awareness, and have provided me with great spiritual support in my upbringing. What would I do without you? Thank you. I love you very much.

All praise be to God, the Father, the Son and the Holy Spirit, the Beginning and the End, without whom nothing ever would be made possible. I wish to thank the Lord Jesus Christ for being my Friend, Saviour and Ruler, and for being within me throughout the time of writing, and forevermore.

No day could ever pass by without you.
I'm so glad that I've found you.
Thank you Jesus.
Thank you King.

Debra Rufini is a woman of many parts: An obsessive, an artist, a thinker, published poet, Kate Bush look–alike, ultra loyal friend.

'Professor Richard Dawkins' Therapy Session with the Wonderful Counsellor' is a work springing from the last in that list of attributes.

Ms. Rufini's friendship with her Creator – along with her fierce loyalty towards that eclectic crowd she numbers among her human friends – addicts, evangelicals, those society terms as 'losers', lovers of God . . . .forms the basis of her new book.

It spans the full spectrum – from the title work, the underlying message of which urges the angry and disappointed Professor to search out and befriend his Creator – to Loopy Lottie, a keenly observed tale of the abnormal. Interspersed are explanations: some Biblical, some autobiographical.

Professor Richard Dawkins' 'Therapy Session'
With the Wonderful Counsellor

The Bible and Debra Rufini have not always sat easily together. Now in her third decade, she's apparently stopped taking issue with the title page of God's communication with His Creation – and ceased fighting His call to friendship. As she says in her dedication: "No day could ever pass by without you . . . . thank you King."

But along with her strongly Creationist message, there are observations on a world gone awry; people – herself? – making mistakes; and – definitely autobiographical – an awakening to theological blindness, in particular with regard to sexuality.

Her closing pieces express a no-holds – barred appreciation of her King – in His time as great as social misfit as Rufini herself has – on occasion – felt.

Debra Rufini is not run-of-the-mill, so this latest publication isn't going to be either. But the author of Social Misfit isn't about to disappoint her readers with anything less than her normal, punchy, pithy, clear-sighted, poetic observations of life, death and God's Universe.

Debra C. Rufini

Professor Richard Dawkins' 'Therapy Session' With the Wonderful Counsellor

Forward

I was inspired to write a short story exploring the possibility of Professor Richard Dawkins seeking therapy, but his 'Wonderful Counsellor' turns out to be the man whom he helped place on the cross!

I first saw Richard Dawkins on the BBC programme 'The Root Of All Evil'. He set out on a mission to convince viewers that Religion was basically evil, and how there couldn't possibly be a God.

Initially I hesitated to watch this, bearing in mind that he is a world-renowned scientist. Would I be persuaded away from my Christian standpoint? What was this 'clever' man clearly seeing that I wasn't? Could it possibly be that I could clearly see something that he couldn't? Surely not! Bravely, I fearfully tuned in. To my absolute astonishment as the broadcast progressed, I realised that the latter was the case!

His aggression was apparent throughout. Was this indeed his 'root of all disbelief?' In his eyes the points he felt relevant to present us with, such as the 'teapot theory' - supposing a teapot is apparently circling the earth, yet its existence cannot be proved, despite the highest level of faith in this one might hold, along with his burning 'what created God then?' enquiry, I couldn't help but believe that he wasn't really listening to himself?! Could he really not come up with anything more convincing? If this was the Professor's very best effort, no wonder his programme had the reverse effect from his intentions.

I may not have numerous letters after my name, but I at least have my common sense. In comparison, I felt highly qualified!

Looking too far, he was missing the point. Or was he simply not looking far enough?

I have always been intrigued to learn how the atheist mind works.

From the programme I perceived that it doesn't - it assumes:
and with no rational backup at that.
The programme ended.
I breathed a sigh of relief.
My God hadn't been shattered.
I made myself a nice cup of tea.
I felt like a genius!!

1 Professor Richard Dawkins' Therapy Session With The Wonderful Counsellor

"Ah Richard, at last we meet,
let me shake you by the hand.
I understand it's your first time here,
and that it wasn't what you'd planned."
"Thank you Sir for your welcome, I'd been advised
to come.
I'd been informed you were a 'wonderful
counsellor',
so gathered no harm could be done."

"You see, I'm under such stress right now.
Are you at all familiar with my work?
My career sets out to save the deceived.
'The God Delusion' is my book to convert.
Striving to explain to all, to make them all see
sense.
'If this book works as I intend,
then those for God will be against."

"Do you know, there are still those who claim
even in this modern time.
Have you ever heard anything so ridiculous,
that this world demanded design?!
Such deluded people
who believe that a man who died
two thousand odd years ago, still lives
and will return right by their side!"

"Well, it does sound a bit far fetched
Mr. Dawkins, I must agree,

but before we explore any more,
let's explore the possibilities.
Would you like to tell me about your childhood?
How you never got that bike you prayed for,
or how you were misunderstood,
or the only school kid who was poor."

"You strike me as angry, dear man.
Setting out on your mission to disprove.
I wonder how much would rely on disbelief
if only your aggression were removed!
Did you want the bike for Christmas?
How old would you have been?
No, no, Mr. Dawkins, please don't leave.
I can see you're turning green!"

"I fail to understand your temper tantrum
at something you cannot believe."
"What I can't believe is why I came here
for this treatment I'm about to receive!
What created God then?"
"But Mr. Dawkins, what came first?
Does it matter if it were the chicken or the egg?
They both exist through birth."

"Well, what about the teapot theory,
that's circling the earth with no proof.
Holding faith that it's really there does not make it
factual truth."
"Well if the earth were covered in tea,
dripping off its side,
its existence, though not evidence
would indicate a teapot nearby."

"For such a clever man one would assume
that you present me with a better case.
These really are such pointless points
on which they're being based.
I really can't expect you
to find spiritual backup,
when your mind's set to disbelief.
It's too early for me to pack up."

"Where is your inbuilt instinct
to believe, no questions asked?
Demanding all the answers,
the biggest man takes on a task.
Man will never 'discover' God,
not because he's not there,
simply because beyond science lies
the truth that you've tried to tear."

"If you can't fit God into a test tube,
'cos it's just way too small,
if there's no positive result,
then he can't exist at all!
If never there was any life breath
down the line to reach us here today,
then there would still be darkness,
as once there was before God had his say."

"Out of nothing comes nothing,
yet we are something, isn't that true?
Wouldn't you agree, Mr. Dawkins,
or is that in your delusion too?
Another intelligent atheist,
once again with lacking common sense

for their case for atheism,
and at my expense!"

"Tell me, what do you mean by that?
Isn't the counsellor supposed to hear me?
Isn't your job for me to talk,
and to listen to me clearly?"
"Tell me Richard, was it a special bike?
I understand 'choppers' caused a lot of fuss.
You see, if we're not careful,
we become the result of what life has thrown at us!"

"Sit down, sit down - I've clearly touched a nerve.
Why did you feel the need to see me,
when you can obviously do it all in your strength,
or would you now disagree?
There's one thing here that doesn't make sense,
that I just do not understand;
if you believe you are no more than a spec,
if you believe you were unplanned ...."

"So you claim to be of minute existence,
where the massive span of time is involved.
Why then are you ranting & raving
& wasting it on something dissolved?!
Haven't you got a hobby,
a much more fun thing to do?"
"You seem to know so very much about me, Sir,
although I don't agree with you!"

"Now then, what is it your 'delusion' book says,
the one that you attack?
'fool says in his heart there is no God'
no God is fact!"

Professor Richard Dawkins' 'Therapy Session'
With the Wonderful Counsellor

"I need a glass of cordial.
My throat is getting dry.
I'm thirsty yet my hunger
doesn't want to give this flavour a try."

"Well, if you decide to come back to me,
you will never thirst again.
Next time I suggest you put your glasses on,
so you recognise who I am!"
"I'm sorry, Mr. Therapy,
I didn't catch your name."
"Well, that's because you didn't ask,
or listen to my pain."

"Now, how much do I owe you?
I don't feel that you've been of much use,
but I'm prepared to pay you anyway,
(if only to cover any abuse!)"
"You needn't, Mr. Dawkins,
you see, I've already paid.
So let me shake you by the hand,
and hope to see you again.
Hey Richard, if you do decide
to return to me once you've gone,
then I'll make sure that I'll see you through,
oh, and that it's got stabilizers on!!"

Romans Chapter 1, Verses 20 & 21

'For since the creation of the world His invisible
attributes are clearly seen, being understood by the
things that are made, even His eternal power &
Godhead, so that they are without excuse, because
although they knew God, they did not glorify Him as
God, nor were thankful, but became futile in their
thoughts, and their foolish hearts were darkened.'

'The God Delusion' features a quote from Richard
Dawkins, stating that a garden should be beautiful
enough in itself without believing that fairies are at
the bottom of it. Surely if fairies were at the bottom
of the beautiful garden, wouldn't their obvious
question be; "How did we get here? Who put this
amazing garden here? What or who is responsible
for our beautifully crafted wings, along with all these
incredible perfectly formed flowers? Who designed
all of this? This couldn't all have mindlessly
'evolved'!"

The disbelievers have not got a leg to stand on,
because they have not witnessed anything to not
believe in, whereas the believers believe, because
they have witnessed. We must also bear in mind
that improbability is not the same as impossibility.
You only have to look at life itself for that backup of
proof!

It's far fetched enough to believe that human life
evolved on its own accord out of mindless cells, but
how can the complexity of the human mind,
(consisting of conscience, consciousness, diverse

emotions, creativity, memory, intelligence, instinct, decision making etc.) possibly evolve on its own accord out of mindless cells?!

Indeed we haven't merely been designed, but in fact over designed. For instance, humans have hands designed for creative tasks. You do not need the most incredibly structured hands (as we have) purely to throw a spear. Literature, art, music & singing are not skills designed for our survival, but for our pleasure. A designer would intend us to use & appreciate such abilities.

Humans have a personality. Therefore the initiator of that personality must also have personality. An initiator devoid of personality could not be responsible for creating one. The result cannot be more complex than the cause.

Most of us are born with the five senses to detect our surroundings, which we're provided with. Our hunger & thirst are catered for by food & drink. What knew that we needed this in order to survive?

Had planet earth been set any nearer to the sun, we would burn up, or any further from the sun, we would freeze up.
Had planet earth been built larger or smaller, its atmosphere would be one where it would not be possible for us to breathe.

We require the oxygen of plants, just as plants require the carbon dioxide of us.

I must say, this 'big bang' appears to be extremely intelligent – everything in the workings & consistency for the universe all fits together too nicely & conveniently.

It has been said by one scientist, that the concept that life came about through sheer chance is as absurd & improbable as a tornado blowing through a junk yard, consequently assembling a Boeing 747! How very true!
Explosions do not produce order, but rather chaos. We cannot get the highly ordered universe we have from a 'big bang'. Skill is essential to create something, and with time, order goes to chaos. Evolution is the opposite, saying that with time life becomes more ordered.

Scientists in Darwinian times believed that the more science progressed, the more it would discover that life at the bottom would be a simple phenomenon, but with the more scientific research given, the more complex the basis has become.

If in the evolutionist's eye we arrived through random processes, then why in the evolutionist's eye does God demand a Creator? God is eternal, and something which is eternal can neither be created nor destroyed.

It takes more faith to believe that we came about by a series of accidents than to believe that we were created by God – to believe that life began by accident, followed by a series of further accidents, producing all the thousands of different kinds of animals & plants that we have today.

Every missing link that has ever been discovered has eventually been proved to be either man, monkeys or hoaxes.
There are millions of missing links between all species. These are called transitional forms. However, there are no examples of transitional forms that have ever been found & proved valid. There should be billions of examples in the fossil record, yet we have everything fully formed.

We are willing to believe in physically unseen waves that exist through the air, operating physical forces & appliances to work, yet not supernatural God forces being responsible for the same! An explosion & a load of time, consisting of no designer, planner, creator at all?! It has been said that evolution is a fairy tale for adults, sadly, where we cannot live happily ever after!

Matter cannot organise itself. For example, a tomato will not progress on its own accord to form a perfect pineapple. It will transform into mould, into disorganisation. The laws of evolution fall flat!

While it's true that species have the ability to adapt to their environment - (micro evolution), species crossing species barriers, (macro evolution) & evolving into other species is totally false.

If we were to assemble ourselves from atoms, we

wouldn't be alive, but just corpses. The miracle of life can only come from a Creator God.

God has left his fingerprints all over the universe. He is inside & outside of the universe, along with time. He is the Divine Consciousness. God does not merely exist. HE IS EXISTENCE!

2 Science Is Only The Stuff That Man Can Reach!

There has to have been a point in time
where life was breathed into the whole of existence.
Out of nothing comes nothing.
Something enabled life's assistance.
Chemicals clashing,
explosions flashing. They do not have a mind!
A big bang alone can't be responsible for it, can it?!
It's common sense to believe
that we didn't put ourselves on this planet!

We don't want to use this swear word, 'God',
Are we afraid of having to limit him to one fixed
abode?
An energy outside of human existence must exist,
or we would remain in darkness mode,
as was the same
before the explosion of light came.
Does it not make perfect sense?!
It all falls hand in hand in its clear indication.
What more can God do to prove himself,
when we've closed our minds from persuasion?!

If we arrived by chance only,
wouldn't other things happen by chance too?!
Are we mistakes then?
We get freak conditions, but they are few.
Not enough to understand
that we're unplanned.
Other things don't take place by chance.

What knows that the skeleton must grow the same
rate as the flesh?
Our development is mapped.
What knows we have to eat? Food's here by
chance I guess!!

Scientifically, energy can never die.
We are water and dust but also emotion and
memory,
for what the physically seen matter alone
takes no responsibility.
Chemicals clashing,
explosions flashing.
A mind comes behind creation.
There's a whole lot more to life than what we can
humanly see.
There's a whole lot more to life
and to complex you and me!

The reason man will never discover God,
is not because he's not there, but because he's
beyond science.
Just because science can't prove,
we mustn't dismiss life's unfathomed giants!
Can't put love or hate
into a test tube and wait
for its existence in a lab.
Yet we believe in emotion, just as God, we can't
physically detect.
God is before and after science.
Man has much to find within the universe as yet!

We have animals that sense what we cannot
detect.

Professor Richard Dawkins' 'Therapy Session'
With the Wonderful Counsellor

Because we can't see invisible company clear
surrounding us by our human eye,
doesn't mean to say that they're not here!
You say I've been brainwashed into believing
what I believe in, in receiving, but it works both
ways;
Have I been brainwashed with Christianity as much
as you have with psychology?!
Every time you point the finger at me,
three point back at you with no apology!

It's interesting that you don't often hear of atheists
that have experienced the paranormal or
supernatural.
Who have witnessed faith or ghosts.
You cannot disprove another's case that's factual.
There's too much evidence
of supernatural events.
The whole concept of God
and life after death is way beyond wishful flatteries,
but in the majority, an inbuilt common sense.
we leave our shells behind
rather than fizzle out like batteries!

There's too much spiritual backup
for it all to be simply bare.
You're making two and two make seven.
You're not looking at what's blatantly there!
You're looking way ahead.
You're lost where you've been led.
Man has to be the highest.
He demands all the answers, he can't make room
for question marks.

They simply won't do.
But now tell me, what breathed life at the start?!

Things don't enable or create themselves.
We can still have evolved by what the almighty has grown.
The day that man makes a man,
Not reproduces or clones,
but takes the raw ingredients,
and breathes in him obedience,
and forms him as his own,
as Frankenstein's creator, that's the day I panic and surrender,
and become an atheist-
living life as the average contender!

3 All My Surrounding

My existence is my certainty,
as I swim around for days.
I don't know how I got here,
and outside looks pretty vague.
All my surrounding
is contained within this bowl.
This is all I see.
This is all I know.

If I get too near the edge,
I can see within the blur,
there are those who wander freely,
there are caged ones who have fur.
But all my surrounding
is contained within this bowl.
This is what I see.
This is all I know.

I have no concept of the room next door.
I have to neglect the idea that there's more.
Forget telling me that a house holds my seat,
or explaining to me that I live in a street.

My existence is my certainty,
as I live from day to day.
They tell me how I got here,
but the scientists are vague.
All my surrounding
is contained within my planet that's on show.
This is all I see.
This is all we know.

We can peer out from the edge,
and discover there is more.
We are clever in our understanding.
Some understanding isn't sure.
All our surrounding
is contained within our planet that's on show.
This is what we see.
This is all we know.

We have no concept of the universes next door,
but we can't neglect the idea that there's more.
Forget telling me in your knowledge limited,
that an explosion caused this vastness,
and that God never did.

So, if you're a goldfish in a bowl,
or a man who journeys far,
never deny existence of the soul,
or more beyond the furthest star.
Whether you're the man who's reached the moon,
or the lecturer with persistence,
inside & out of it all,
God is its existence.

4 Planet Zoor

A little man from planet Zoor came rushing to his
friends,
to tell that he had been to Earth,
and to let them know our trends.
Well, the Zoorites said;
"He's cracked up now, he's just escaped from his
mind!"
So little Zoorlot wandered home,
and hoped one day that they'd find.
"They've got these beings called 'people' there,
they have two arms and legs".
But they just didn't believe or care.
"They've only got one head", he said.
"They also have these objects which fly.
I think they're called aeroplanes.
They go real high up in the sky.
They've also got computer games".
The Zoorites laughed and laughed once more,
as poor old Zoorlot claimed;
that if he was in their shoes right then,
he would have done the same.
"How I wish I could take you there,
but I don't know the way.
I wish you could see these humans,
it's so funny how they play".

Well, they don't believe,
because their minds can't accept.
They're brought up in that way.
They don't know any differently.
They're not us.

And that's the way it may always stay.
"It's a fairy tale", they say.
There must be a much bigger being
to create them in that way.
What they don't realise is that humans made them
up from far away.
"We're one step higher from them", we say.

Do you believe me when I say that a man will come
from the sky,
and only take the ones who love him
to live with him way up high?
Well, you may say that I've cracked up now,
and I've just escaped from my mind!
So now I'll just wander back home,
and hope one day that you'll find.
They've got these beings called 'angels' there.
They're clad in white and have wings.
But you just don't believe or care.
They've even got a voice which sings.
They worship too the one in the sky.
The one who I said will come.
Why waste your time on wondering why,
when you can get to know the Son?
The humans laughed and laughed once more,
as poor old I still claim;
that if I was in their shoes right then,
I would have made a change.
How I wish I could take you there,
but for you I don't know the way.
I wish you could see what I see,
because it's so sad the way you play.

Well, they don't believe,

because their minds can't accept.
They're brought up in that way.
They don't know any differently.
We're not God,
and that's the way it will always stay.
So, "it's a fairy tale", they say.
There surely must be a much bigger being to make
us in this way.
What some don't realise is that our Creator
made us up from far away.
"He's one step higher from us", I say.

5 "I'm Sorry Son"

"Yes, this is good, I'm satisfied with my creation.
I think these things I've made are right where
they're stood,
 but I need more to make a population,
not just plants, birds and wood.
I'll build a man, and show him what a life is.
I'll take a rib from him,
and show him what a wife is.
I'll build his perfect wife,
then they shall start to raise the nation,
all living perfect lives."

"My work is done,
of building Adam's wife, Eve.
They live so happily,
so free and have fun,
but what's all this;
hiding behind my bushes.
Why from me do they run?
In Eve's hand I see that poisonous fruit,
I told her not to pick.
She disobeyed my voice,
but she was told by my only enemy,
to go ahead by choice."

"I'm sorry, then,
it's too late, I said not to.
You disobeyed my word,
my one strict command,
and now your sons follow by your example.
Sin, they now understand.
One Son is dead,

by murder of his brother,
so from now on we'll have wrong things passed on
through life.
The only way to gain them back,
is to give my only Jesus Christ."

"I'm sorry, Son,
you have to save my people.
They've all gone their own way,
because of what Eve has done.
I'm sending you,
but only because I need to,
though you're the perfect one.
You'll never sin, instead take it from others.
When you die on a cross you'll carry their sin
weight.
The only way to bring them back to me is,
by them entering your gate"

"Oh, Father dear,
I'm down here doing your will.
I have twelve men with me,
they always stay near,
and they believe, and see and know what I feel.
They know what I'm doing here.
Many people believe I'm from the Devil.
When I claim that I am yours,
some can get real angry.
The other day they gave me such a cold chill,
when they didn't see you in me."

"They need me here,
to get to you, my Father,

but they just don't believe your words in their ear.
They want me dead.
They say that I am a liar,
Yet I shall never fear
I hear them say,
'Who does this man think he is?'
while others follow me and cling on to your word.
I feel the time for me to arrive faster,
to you has come I heard."

"Oh, God don't go,
I feel so much agony.
I feel the pain of their sin weigh in me so low.
Yet they all laugh.
Those soldiers blinded, can't see.
Hopefully they will know.
Accept me now,
and this guy with me also.
I can't wait to move on to help prepare your place.
It is finished.
The curtain rips, and I see the changed mood on
their face."

"Truly this man
 was the Son of the highest."
The miracles performed, I'll never understand.
When once they thought
 the man was such a true fake,
 ruining our land.
And so today,
I'll leave you with this story.
Hope you don't find yourself in the soldiers' same
case,
but if you do,

remember that the greatest died for you in your
place.

So if you come,
and ask our dear Lord Jesus,
to take your sins on him and make you see the sun,
then you won't go,
when the time runs out in your life,
to the place where you can't run.
It never ends,
eternal burning torture,
but we've been freed from that,
and you don't have to go.
Instead we have a saviour who can free us,
by giving him your soul.

6 The Time Of God signs

Oh, man he is so clever.
He can forecast all the weather,
and see when it's gonna rain,
and if there's a disturbance in a function,
he's observant,
to cure the right kind of pain.
Dinosaur bones and danger zones,
he's fully made aware,
but he won't take a look,
in the common sense book,
still with all the knowledge he bears.
He's blunt to the time of God signs.
With all of his knowledge,
that's still way out from his mind.
The time of God signs.
To never believe that God's judgement is nigh.
Will never believe in the time of God signs.

Only knows up to his limit,
of cleverness that's within it,
and tries to fathom the unexplained.
The only parts that we're meant to understand,
well, that's not enough for this big man,
so he throws the whole lot away.
For not fathoming out,
he gives up, so doubts,
so according to man,
it's untrue.
So, alters to man's level of believing,
hence, the real truth, not receiving.
Doesn't know that this baffling God is watching him
too.

Professor Richard Dawkins' 'Therapy Session'
With the Wonderful Counsellor

He's well and truly blunt to the time of God signs.
With all of his mystery guessing,
the truth is still way out from his mind.
The time of God signs.
Will never accept that mystery God is mysteriously
high.
Will never believe in the time of God signs.

7 The End Of Time Signs

Signs are here to warn us,
that nigh is coming upon us,
God's earth to a final stand still.
Earthquakes, hurricanes and famines.
All these we can examine,
and come up with a reason to God's works kill.
Man still running.
The end nearer coming.
He sits in the corner and hides.
Probably scared, but never aware,
that safe is on God's side.
He's blunt to the end of time signs.
With all his fearing,
that's still a blot out from his mind.
The end of time signs.
To always forget that the time will soon be nigh.
Will never believe the end of time signs.

Uses man to give men warnings,
and is unto them calling.
Even though man is unaware.
T.V. cameras at the situations,
to broadcast to all the nations,
that if not saved; The daunting scare.
But just as man, he doesn't know,
that God is using him to show.
Man is quite unaware too,
of what these warnings mean.
To him, they're just yet another disaster upon the
screen,
 blamed on God by me and you.
He's blunt to the end of time signs.

Professor Richard Dawkins' 'Therapy Session'
With the Wonderful Counsellor

With all his fearing,
that's still a blot out from his mind.
The end of time signs.
Will never cling onto;
God moves in mysterious ways.
Will never accept that these are the end of time
signs.

You say that we've been saying that for years.
Trying to put in you the fear,
but nothing's happened as yet.
Well, the world's not getting better.
People can't prolong it forever.
It has to be God met.
The longer we're sat here waiting,
the longer we're hesitating,
to let it slip from our hands.
No, we can't keep up what's given,
and forever we can't live in,
this flesh destiny or residence of God's plan.
So let's be aware of the end of time signs,
and in it have salvation non-fearing,
for a certain peace of mind.
The end of time signs.
Let's always be aware,
that the time will soon be nigh,
and always believe that now are the end of time
signs.

8 A Mass Flight Into Space
(Last Piece Of The Puzzle)

God light surrounding to glow
the chosen few that you should know.
Cupped by hands, together bound.
The unbelievers' vision scoffs.
Doubter hanging on the edge
of the hand destined to pledge.
Climbs onto the finger small,
only to be shaken off.

Earth not as yet seen the last
let alone the first, peeked by the vast.
The final view of Jesus Christ
will not be one in weakness.
A reversal in this picture concerned.
Piercings of strength hold his return,
not as Saviour this time around,
rather as the Ruler crowned.

The world's biggest sensation
beamed on every TV station.
'The Missing Millions' reads headline.
One to firmly pitch us.
How the world will then respond;
"We don't quite know what happened,
but their common factor stands;
they were all 'religious'!"

Sceptic scoffers forever humming;
"Where's the promise of his coming?"
God's gracious plan of love vows
to be perfect and honest.

Professor Richard Dawkins' 'Therapy Session'
With the Wonderful Counsellor

Lengthening out the day of grace,
unwilling that any should perish and waste,
but all would come to repentance.
Not slack in concerning his promise.

Prophecy is the Bible's proof
that the Bible is the truth.
Certainty is guaranteed
in the Holy Scripture.
What the 'high' books have to say,
how the influences stray,
education disobeys,
to distort the clearest picture.

His Majesty's second advent
is mentioned more than when first sent.
The day lies hid, that every day
we be watchful and wise.
Living each day like it were
when his return will occur.
Keeping us Holy and to
urgently evangelise.

Like a thief he'll arrive, (our sin slave),
robbing the world of its saved,
like a big surprise unannounced,
while the world is sleeping.
Totally casual, totally unprepared,
a world troubled by tragic affairs,
but the last thing on its mind
will be this visitor's greeting.

What a mess he'll come back to clear out.

No wonder he's coming with a shout.
Many will jump from not hearing about
this momentous occasion.
Drugging themselves into oblivion,
losing what they could have won,
leaving salvation undone
to face this dreadful invasion.

Light and salt gone, Hell let loose.
Mark of the Beast introduced.
We now have technology
to track every person.
Those who took this Christ to receive,
further than history's fact believed,
have escaped found,
but the lost have escaped God's version.

In the twinkling of an eye,
into space this mass will fly
with him, and I will deny
this as an unlikely story.
Alone, this ship world would not float,
but thank God Christ's the lifeboat.
Thank God, death is swallowed up
in this great victory.

The plot currently incomplete,
awaiting the rest to take its seat.
The second arrival paints
the whole picture clearly.
The Earth must cease its beating heart,
to begin eternity's start.
If Satan reminds you of your past,
remind him that his future's dreary!

9 It's Only Heathen Nature

Mr. Heathen nature,
he goes to bed.
He hears the sound of the loud planes up ahead.
"Oh no, what if it's now the end of the world?"
is his worry.
God suddenly appears from nowhere in his life.
For the very first time he is real.
"I'm not ready yet."
So what can be done in such a hurry?
The planes pass by,
and no more is heard his worrying cry.
Then God suddenly vanishes into thin air.
So to carry on with another normal day to bear.

Mr. Heathen nature,
next day the same.
He hears the big storm and the almighty roars of
the wind and the rain.
"Oh no, what if this time is really the end of the
world?"
Is his worry.
God suddenly appears again from nowhere in his
life.
For the second time he is real.
"I'm not ready yet."
So just what can be done in such a hurry?
The storm quickly passes by,
and no more is heard the sound of his trembling
cry.
Then God suddenly vanishes into thin air.
So to carry on with another normal day to bear.

Mr. Heathen nature,
at the wake of the dawning,
he hears the fake sound of the three minute
warning.
"Oh no, what if this is really the end of the world?"
Is about all that's within his worry.
God suddenly appears again from nowhere in his
life.
For the third time he is real.
"I'm not ready yet."
So what can be done in such a hurry?
The warning shortly passes by,
and no more is heard the sound of his worrying cry.
Then God once again vanishes into thin air.
Just how many normal days are left and faced to
bear?

But, oh Mr. Heathen nature,
when all of these false warnings have passed,
you don't know how many more are in store for
sure,
but will you be ready when the final trumpet sounds
its blast?
Mr. Heathen nature,
you are strong when the living is at its norm.,
but you are trembling at the sight of the unexpected
storm.
This is when you have to test your soul.
What else can human life turn to?
You don't look ahead prepared for the next
surprise.
The next one could be all too late for you.
Total confidence in yourself in everyday living,

can control all of these until a major crisis is
winning.

Mr. Heathen nature,
next day is Christ's return.
It's much too late now for all that rubbish
 you once learnt.
"Oh no, it looks like this is really the end of the
world."
Is all that's concerned in his worry.
God suddenly appears again visible this time in his
life.
For the fourth time this time in his life he is real.
"I'm not ready yet."
But it's too late now,
so don't even attempt to hurry.
The Lord passes by,
and evermore is heard his worrying cry.
Then God suddenly vanishes into thin air.
Never another God to call for,
in his eternal lonely fears to bear.

10 Saved, But Sad Hurt Eyes

He was genuine.
He requested Jesus in,
at the age of sweet sixteen.
He knew how it was to be,
a born again in thee,
and he knew how his soul was clean.
He would help the needy,
and witness to the dying.
Then he would rush off home,
to watch 'The life of Brian'

He's staring in the saved,
but sad hurt eyes.
The anguish of his Lord sees no surprise.
So caring and carrying in all his tasks,
 yet he's wearing a mask.

He worships day and night,
and he is the first to fight
the opinions of all those who don't believe.
He's the most encouraging,
but the most blaspheming.
Just from which side does he receive?
He will preach for hours from the book of
Revelation,
and rush home from the meeting to watch 'The last
temptation'.

When the last trumpet will sound,
will he look all around, and laugh;
"Jesus, look who's here!"
When the gates let him in,

Professor Richard Dawkins' 'Therapy Session'
With the Wonderful Counsellor

through that gap in his sin,
what kind of humour then will appear?
Will guiltiness at last be recognised by these
sights?
The ones that he should have known.
Will he view a different picture this time
when he heads off for home?

How can you take part in the Holy Communion,
and then return to your wicked and back-stabbing
reunion?

I was aware from an early age that I had a physical attraction towards my own gender. Without paying too much attention to the matter at the time, as time went on I soon began to realise that being actively gay wasn't right, so never acted on my tendancy. Being brought up in a Christian home gave me a moral foundation. I had a handful of short-term relationships with guys, but there always seemed to be something missing, so I consequently put into action my 'natural persuasion'.

'Coming out' as it were, and being very much involved in the gay scene, I was able to express myself and have the relationships that I wanted. I had previously given my life to the Lord in my teens, but at the age of twenty two I felt that it was time to please ME for a change, so I left God behind. The gay scene was fun, exciting. I was continuously searching for Miss right, and in the process receiving pain upon pain and rejection upon rejection. The gay scene generally is what's best described as a meat market, and revolves around sex that people mistake for pure love & inner fulfilment. There is much heartache to be found in these places. Incredibly lively venues filled with laughter & happy faces, yet they are the loneliest of places. A typical sight on a Saturday night outside the club would be one of couples fighting, shouting, or someone storming out in tears. Everyone here is looking for something that nobody seems to find! Although I never personally became involved in such activities, my surrounding soon became one of drug taking, prostitution, rape, cruising and the like. Every few weeks at the club we would hear of the latest guy who had become HIV infected. This was normality! For example; a group of men sharing a syringe with the attitude of "It doesn't matter, 'cos we've all got it!"

Then one day I met an Italian man in one of the pubs. We got talking and discovered that we were as empty and unfulfilled as each other, with failed after failed same sex relationship, so we consequently got married. It seemed like a good idea at the time! Our marriage lasted for six long years, until we both came to the conclusion that we were unhappy and denying ourselves of who we were, so we divorced and it was back to square one for us.

Which route was there left for us? I'd tried the right way – celibate by God, the wrong way – actively gay, without God. Could I possibly be actively gay with Jesus as my Lord? And so I explored the possibility. The Metropolitan Community Church (MCC) was advertised in the 'Gay Times' monthly. For a church to exist, combining God with allowing me to be who I am, they must surely have some Biblical justification for this. If this were the case, I was not prepared to live a life which wasn't ideal for me, if the two could live in harmony. I attended both Portsmouth & Bournemouth branches for roughly two years, but the more I tried to educate myself & reasure myself with their 'wishy washy' school of thought, the more apparent it became to me that their justification for homosexuality in practise being alongside Biblical teaching was just so ridiculous.

The MCC newsletter features a page which reads; 'Gay, straight, bisexual, transgendered, transvestite – God loves us all.' This indeed couldn't be nearer to the truth, but it failed to recognise that God's love & God's approval are very much not the same thing. A large part of their thinking rests on Jesus himself not saying anything against it. This is typical of what you can expect to read on banners held high at a gay pride march; - 'This is what Jesus had to say about homosexuality' –

....
....They totally ignore that Jesus' teaching was very much in favour of the stability of family life. Anything that is mentioned in the Old Testament about it, they shrug it off as irrelevant old Jewish law, & in Romans where we're told it's 'unnatural', they will claim that 'unnatural' doesn't mean 'wrong'. I knew in my heart that they were making two & two make seven. For me, Genesis is the book that we cannot go against or get away from. Right at the start of God's word, we're told that God would make a helper suitable for man, (and it wasn't in the form of another man!) As much as I really didn't want to come to this conclusion, it was now time for me to stop fighting against God's truth. As much as I could shake my fist in the air and throw a tantrum at God, I knew that I just couldn't beat God or change His mind on the issue.

During this time, whilst still attending both churches, I had problems with anxiety and subsequent chest pain. One day, I was with my parents having a cup of tea in a café, when I felt very ill. I came outside, collapsed on the floor, and was whisked away by ambulance with a suspected heart attack. As I lay there in pain, wired up, gaze fixed on the ECG monitor, it dawned on me - "if that line goes straight, (and I haven't been,) I've had it, and I won't make it to Heaven." The experience in the ambulance taught me so many things. I promised God there and then that I would never return to either church, or sleep with another woman. I repeated the prayer of repentance (and meant it this time!) I spent the next few days with my parents. I decided to cut myself off from certain people who would hinder my growth in the Lord. I learnt so much in those few days of rest than ever before – 'how could I claim to love God, whilst doing something he detests?' Rather than it being a case of 'what has God got planned for me in order to prosper me?' it was a matter of 'how much can I get away with?!' Whenever I was in the (gay) club or in church, I used to pray "Lord, please don't return tonight!"

At the time, I became fascinated with atheist, Professor Richard Dawkins, and kept reminding myself; 'if we are the product of random, mindless evolution, then it really doesn't matter what gender (or even species) goes with who, but if we are the result of planned creation, then it can't possibly be by chance that the complexity of the male and the female bodies are so obviously designed to compliment each other.

This topic is controversial. It saddens me when churches take a 'liberal' view in the 'anything goes' attitude. God is never changing. He doesn't change His laws for anyone, even though man may legalise to suit him. It also saddens me when Christians (sometimes unaware that they're doing so,) target homosexuality as the sin above all sins. I think there is a tendency when something doesn't concern us, or if it's something that we don't understand, we can wrongly assume that it's a worse sin than the next. We must remind ourselves that a gay person is not of that persuasion by choice, and it is often very much a struggle for them to live that way, even more so a struggle to pull away from what is 'naturally' felt.

Many gay people loathe God (or the idea of God,) because they believe that God loathes them (as people.) Many cannot distinguish between their actions and themselves. We are far more than our sexuality – we are all equally loved by God, and the gay person needs to be told this, as much as we need to love them, whilst not condoning their actions.

11 Once Upon A Time

"Huh, daughters eh, they think they know what's
best.
She grabbed the rib, and grabbed the fruit, grabbed
you
and grabbed all the rest!"
"Hello Debra, nice to meet you,
haven't we met before?
Can I tempt you with one of these,
before I bake some more?"
"You and your wretched treats, woman,
has gone on way too far.
Ooh, look at that bit with icing on,
        um no thanks, but ta!"

Once upon a time there was a girl.
She took the rib and the fruit and the bliss.
"Hmmm, now what can I make out of all of this?"
she thought.
No use remembering what she was taught.
"Could make a crumble or a cage, I guess,
but where's the fun in that?
No, I'll simply make a mess!
So is this how it was meant to be?
This woman for you and this man for me?"
So she lived, and she danced,
and she cried, and she died.
And we must never forget the fact that she tried.

Once upon a time
there was a girl.
She took the plunge in her search to agree.

She knew how it wasn't meant to be.
She took the rib and the fruit and the bliss.
"Hmmm, now what can I make out of all of this?"
she thought.
No use remembering what she was taught.
"God works in mysterious ways -
the know all killjoy who works for the best.
Take this man with whom you are blessed!
Well, my heart's filled with pride ..... dig deep, dig
deep.
I share in your loss, Miss Little Bo Peep!
Wow, if I were attached to Jan Pearson.
We can't keep it up forever, dear boy.
The alternative looks pretty grim, pretty fearsome."

"This seems like it's a safe place to be.
Yum yum, stop stop, you're sat next to matrimony.
Look straight ahead, pay attention to the guy.
This is what you've come here for -
to give clear conscience yet another try.
Some people see someone,
and instinct knows they're the only one,
yet don't know or understand why.
God works in mysterious ways.
It's just as well it ain't mutual,
you see it lets me off the hook.
So you see God, in your infinite wisdom,
it's not as it might look.
Yet I'm stabbed through the heart with a red hot
poker.
Slap her or snog her, or try to provoke her.
But the girl at the start was taken from the rib.
Where does this leave us, boy?
Surely God wouldn't fib!"

Professor Richard Dawkins' 'Therapy Session'
With the Wonderful Counsellor

So one day she died,
died inside, died in pride.
And stood before God,
although she wanted to hide.
And he said;
"Well done in doing what you knew you
 had to do.
Just remember that I'm all forgiving,
so I'll let you go through.
Here's someone you'll get on well with
like you would not believe –
meet my 2nd attempt at perfection,
meet my daughter, Eve."

As a young girl at my parents' church, a middle aged woman used to sit with my mother and I. I was curious about her. She never seemed to be as joyous and as full of the spirit of God as the rest of the congregation. She appeared very vacant and starey. What was different about her? Even as a child you can always sense when 'grown ups' aren't good with kids, right? I remember smiling up at her, and gaining lack of response in return.

Then one day I came home from school, when my mother informed me that the lady who sat with us each Sunday at church was very sad, so she decided that she wanted to go and live with Jesus. I was upset, but I didn't show it. Wow, she'd killed herself. How awful. How brave. How I still wish that things had been so very different for such a sweet, yet distant and disturbed woman.

My childhood was a happy one. I had parents and a sister that couldn't be beaten. Yet school life was horrid! I was hardly the height of fashion, I was overweight and so I couldn't relate to or seek the approval of either gender. I still believe that this was part of what contributed to my struggle with same-sex attraction in both childhood and adulthood.

The bullying continued all throughout the school years and as I believe, well into adulthood. It manifested itself into wherever I passed people by in the street or was in a public place, if ever I saw them laughing, whispering, looking my way, I would assume that it was all about mocking me. This eventually got so out of hand, it reached the point that I would approach people wherever I was, wherever they were. I embarrassed them more than I embarrassed myself, whether I had been mistaken in my estimations or not. I received both surprising and baffled responses, as you can well imagine.

There were days when I couldn't function properly, to the point where it became impossible for me to post a letter up the road, or to put my rubbish out. Most of the time I was plastering over the root of the problem with diazepam. Ah yes, thank God for diazepam!

It was my 30th birthday. My parents had arranged a meal at their place with some guests for me. During that day I had gone for a spin in the country with my husband. Two young lads were crossing the zebra crossing, looked in the direction of our car, laughed and carried on walking. I came home, tired, hurt, wanting to escape life – I just couldn't take this yet another time. This treatment would never leave me. This would carry on life long. The only way that I could get a break from it would be to turn to diazepam, (lovely diazepam) and a bottle of red. I failed to make it to my birthday meal, but did make it successfully to the A&E department in the local hospital.

I now knew where my fascinating friend was at – this lovely quiet lady in the church so long ago. But she had made it to the grave. How much more mental pain she must have endured than I. That was pretty much hard to believe, yet it must have been true, even though she'd held it all within.

In the duration spent working for the Samaritans, along with my own personal experience, mental health has taught me many things. A broken limb is visually evident, yet mental torture isn't, so consequently dismissed and ignored many a time. Sometimes we don't recognise it in someone, until we witness the result of it in their death. Never underestimate or belittle depression. It's very real indeed, but there is always help, and there is always a different route that can be taken other than opting out of life. Depression must never triumph. Life is God's precious gift to us, his children. He wants it to be enjoyed by us and for it to be lived to its fullness for the glory of him, our Creator, our loving Father with wide open welcoming arms.

12 Thelma Fews

A Church's fond memory of tragedy seems rare.
"He will not beyond us that limit to bear".
A Mother, a Daughter, an Actress's smile,
sat in the back pew for only a while.
A Mother, a Daughter, a Wife,
shared in a role of all three.
A time to be selfish,
to be spared for the desperation key.

A child so observant could sense the tense strain,
although the undeveloped cannot place their finger
on pain.
Grown ups were supposed to be happy and full of
the cross.
Not vacant and starey, like she always was.
Grown ups were supposed to be happy and
blessed, even in their loss.
Her lacking in something, her life did it cost.

Now, I thought that you had to always put on the
lid,
and pull down the blinds, when this foreigner hit.
And I thought the done thing was for grown ups to
hide,
should a face ever appear absent in having Jesus
at its side.

What does it take to reach for that state of mind,
of kissing the grave, and wishing for closing time?
Differing tragedies all amount to the same.
Their level in sickness doesn't alter the pain.

Debra C. Rufini

Candyfloss life is for only the dense.
Razors are given to those experienced.

Thelma, it's not until now that I understand.
The years have passed by, and I see now life's
plan.
Thelma, I know that your Master within,
has taken you back for REAL life to begin.

So, in her life now, I believe that she's free,
from troubles and muddles and overall catastrophe.
How I wish that I could have saved your suicide.
My age and your mind were not enough to be
applied.
So Thelma, I look forward to meeting with you.
I'm sorry I misunderstood back in the pew.

13 Eccentric Old Bid (Loopy Lottie)

Many claim that she's lost it,
with her ideas that don't fit
their so-called 'normality'.
 A lonely outcast's the outcome –
named 'Loopy Lottie', the odd one.
They're scared to peep outside of sanity.

Her presentation may seem strange.
Her manic grey hair forms a long mane.
Her red shoes are too big for her feet.
Green socks and on her hat, flowers.
They stand laughing at her for hours.
Their amusement act is incomplete.

Since a child, she's been rejected.
Now, old age only wants to be accepted.
She's not asking for as much as to be liked.
Even adulthood faces mockery;
"Something I thought by now would have
left me,
but no, it's clinging on with all its might".

She shouts it out in the High Street;
"I'm mad, and you're sat in my seat",
as they cross over to the other side.
As the centre of their attention,
she doesn't care much for prevention.
She's happy for them to stare with mouths
and eyes wide.

They play their least part to support her.

This neighbourhood disturbed would much
rather abort her.
Can't they see their entertainment needs to
give help a try?
"This world will shrink thin and I'll grow
wide,
then I will leave by jumping off its side",
she yells, as they fail to grasp how the
problem with them lies!

14 Sometimes It Takes

Sometimes it takes
such a massive great mistake,
for someone to see,
or to become the good hearted.
It may have to be
in the form of a tragedy,
in order for them to now appreciate
what they before took for granted.

Sometimes it takes
a gust of wind or an earthquake,
to see things differently,
or to become a better person,
to open closed eyes,
or wake up to realise.
A situation needs to take its place
to teach a lesson in a different version.

At first you may get
a gentle whisper in the head,
then a small gale,
then a hurricane full-blown.
How long will we wait,
until we choose which one to take?
While matters increase and worsen,
how many danger signals must be shown?

Where will we choose
to step off, before the blown fuse?
In life's such hazards,
if we can help them, then let's halt them.

The longer the loose brick lies around,
the sooner the whole house will fall down.
I'd rather catch the subtle breeze's warning,
but maybe for some, that's not enough that's taught
them.

Alec Alcoholic
didn't stop at gin and tonic.
His warning light had flashed blindingly
in his early stages.
It had to take one drink more
before it hit home with the score.
And sooner than he knew it,
he was pushing up the daisies.

Susie Sleeparound
frequently stepped on danger ground.
Her attention wasn't caught.
To the AIDS scare, she didn't listen.
One HIV,
another two, another three.
How many more increased chances should it take
for her to be frightened out of her position?

15 Dear Jeevis

It was ever such a lovely day,
In that rural place so far away.
The family Jeevis with their servant, Grace,
on their tour around to check out the sights of this
place.

Was very cosy, yet not very used to.
They were almost human for once.
There was no such show, for it was only those few,
away from society of the upper kind.
For just one moment in time they left all falseness
behind.

A family nearby, as they always do,
came up to greet the ones who appeared to be
new.
Should the Jeevis family now act above, to show
just who they are?
They were now faced with paupers, who were the
lowest here by far.

The snobbery at first got in the way,
but it wasn't long before they could cope with their
kind of day.
They soon became the closest of the friendship
kind.
After all, they were only the visitors having to leave
offishness behind.

The children play, while the adults talk & natter.

Yes, they were human too, despite their lack of grammar.
They went out, they stayed in, their house became their home.
They accepted every condition & not once did they moan.

Taking to their lifestyle of dirt & sweat.
Well after all, a holiday must be adaptably met.
The Jeevises not too familiar with the surroundings here,
consequently found father Jeevis sinking into a bog too near.
The Jeevises like at almost any other time,
had to go on ahead, leaving the paupers way behind.
They all pulled away not attempting to get
Mr Jeevis out – too busy being upset.

The waiting for the pauper family,
was only a matter of ten seconds preciously to see.
They came running, & they knew exactly what to do,
as they went on ahead & rescued him, unlike the spectating few.

Well, the fun seemed so endless that was enjoyed by them all,
but the time came all too soon for their returning call.
They agreed to communicating about their friendly terms,
but there was one lesson here that the Jeevises should have learnt.

Professor Richard Dawkins' 'Therapy Session'
With the Wonderful Counsellor

Back to the scene of snobbery & inhuman acts.
The family to their true lifestyle were now brought
back.
The adults talk in the upper fashion,
while the children play with no sticks or stones, but
with some toys of action.

All was soon forgotten of their holiday.
They never told any of their friends. Well they were
only paupers anyway.
To the other side, it was their highlight of life,
to have such visitors come to see them there in
their light.

The Jeevis's ball was to take its place,
on an evening so cool with nothing to disgrace.
What incident could ruin such a happy time?
Not a knock at the door, with some peasants
behind.

A face should have seen such a welcome sight,
but instead of which, met with a "go back" bite.
After pleading with the butler to let them come in.
After succeeding in telling their friendship with the
Jeevises was convincing.

"Mr Jeevis", a cry came to halt
all that was going on, as he stopped all to talk.
Astonished gasps filled the air, as the peasant man
saw only their same level now, he could not
understand.

"Won't you let us in & won't you let us stay?

We've suffered a forest fire, which has blown our
house away.
We won't cause you any trouble, that I promise
you,
as you never in our house, which once stood well &
true."

What other statement could turn such upper heads,
as the Jeevis household, embarrassed, but
furiously said:
"Master Grace, please escort these dear people to
the door,"
along with the glare of 'please don't come & visit
here any more!'

How could such a man turn such an incident away?
How could Grace, who became a pal also, know
just what he could say?
They saved his life, gave them a home & freedom
for a while,
but due only to the upper friend's thoughts, had he
to turn so vile.

So they roamed hungry & cold, & with nowhere to
lie.
When one day announced that family pauper had
to die.
They could not go back, so they stayed in that
town's rich face,
where the Jeevis mansion could, but did not offer a
place.

When the bulletin of the family hit the news,
there was only one guilty family to accuse.

Witnesses from the party came forward to declare,
that the family once knew the Jeevis name, for they
were there.

Every Jeevis member went to visit the scruffy
morgue,
In that old shanty town where they had visited once
before.
Looks were upon their dead faces as if to say but
not to moan,
"We'd invite you back for coffee, but we haven't got
a home."

16 King Social Misfit

I've never seen you,
but I've heard you've declared;
"You do it for me,
if for your brother you've cared."
You were an outcast
so many years ago.
You were born poor,
yet with gold, your house glows.
We worship a man 2,000 years gone by,
who the 'religious' rejected & despised.
We avoid in the pew
the man with the smell & the stains.
Would we touch the hem of YOUR garment,
if it appeared the same?!

I've never touched you,
yet you touched people who were untouchable,
and you loved people,
those classed unlovable.
Has your church moved on?!
We shun with lacking embrace,
where acceptance
needs to be the case.
What's gone so wrong,
that's failed to get right?
What would we see
if we could judge YOU by sight?!
You stood up for those
whose actions you could not condone.
King Social Misfit
now sits upon a throne!

Professor Richard Dawkins' 'Therapy Session'
With the Wonderful Counsellor

17 Reaching To My Soul

Thrown into existence,
into infinite room.
You knew my name from your beginning.
You knew my life beyond the womb.
As you sent the rain
to kick start the world again,
so you rinsed me thoroughly,
flooding me, completing me.

Your birth taught us how to live,
to be righteous and true.
It taught me how to love.
Taught me how to be like you.
Preaching your ministry,
how you surely rocked the boat.
Reaching to my soul,
how you surely made me whole.

To the masses, loaves and fish,
you fed with miracle and prayer.
Quenching my thirst, feeding me full,
I know you were really there.
When you calmed the storm
from my life which was shipwrecked,
you tossed away the battling waves.
I was lost this way, but Jesus saves.

Your death conquered the sin,
conquered the death, conquered the stains.
You broke free from your tomb.
I broke free from my chains.

Debra C. Rufini

Every man who dies his death
refusing denial of your truth,
stands by your eternal reign,
longing to meet with you again.

Conclusion

Some well-known atheists of their time had their perceptions changed from what they had previously believed, acknowledging that their lives were an empty existence in a Godless world, living dissatisfied.

They include:-
H.G. Wells, writer (1866 – 1946),
George Bernard Shaw, playwright (1856 – 1950),
Bertrand Russell, British philosopher, mathematician, social critic, writer (1872 –1970). After being asked if he would be prepared to die for what he believed in, he replied; "Of course not, after all, I may be wrong!"
Professor Joad, British philosopher, writer, broadcaster, initially a rationalist. He later had a religious conversion.
Antony Flew, British philosophy Professor. At 81, he had changed his mind, believing that a higher existence must have been responsible for the Universe.

The French philosopher, Voltaire, claimed that 100 years after his death his work would be read, turning people to his writings, as opposed to the Bible: that the Bible would be obsolete. He had wrecked the faith of many. Voltaire died in 1728, yet the Bible continues to live. Ironically, 50 years after his death, his previous house became the Geneva Bible Society, where his printing equipment was used to produce Bibles in their thousands!

Even our 'inventor' of evolution, Mr. Charles Darwin had this to say to Lady Hope when he was almost bedridden for 3 months before he died; "I was a young man with unfathomed ideas. I threw out queries, suggestions, wondering all the time over everything, and to my astonishment the ideas took like wildfire – people made a religion of them." Darwin then asked Lady Hope to speak to neighbours the next day. "What shall I speak about?" She asked. He replied; "Christ Jesus and his salvation. Is that not the best theme?"

In retrospect, one can't help wonder how Professor Dawkin's autobiography will read when he breathes his last. Let us hope and pray that he follows in some of his forefathers footsteps, and that he returns to his 'Wonderful Counsellor'!

So, why the importance where & who we came from? Once you recognise that you are the result of purposeful plan, and not the outcome of accidental chance, then you can begin to plan where you're going to spend eternity.

After all, if God does exist and loves us, He would reveal Himself to us: indeed He has – through His Son, Jesus Christ. He wants us to respond individually to His call to receive Him into our lives, and forgive us our sins, through our repentance of them. Through Jesus' sacrifice – an horrific death on a torturous cross, we can enter into the relationship His Father, God, originally intended for us. All we have to do is ask, receive, and live by His prosperous plan that He has for each and every one of us, His creation. We have this provided for us in His word, the Bible.

John Chapter 3, Verse 16
"For God so loved the world that He gave His only begotten Son,
That whoever believes in Him shall not perish but have eternal life."

18 Life Will Always Cease Us

Life will always cease us to the bone.
It's a game that some will win to lose,
if it's to be played on your own.
So if they question you upon its meaning,
turn to answer them in depth,
that the only one who gave it,
is the only one to save it,
and claim it back when it's been ship-wrecked.